OLIVIA RODRIGO LINES TO LIVE BY

POP PRESS

Pop Press, an imprint of Ebury Publishing
20 Vauxhall Bridge Road
London SW1V 2SA

Pop Press is part of the Penguin Random House group of companies
whose addresses can be found at global.penguinrandomhouse.com

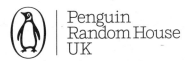

Penguin
Random House
UK

First published by Pop Press in 2024

Design: Jonathan Baker
Text: Becky Alexander
Illustrations: Ollie Mann

www.penguin.co.uk

A CIP catalogue record for this book is available from the British Library

ISBN: 9781529937930

Typeset in 13/15pt Rotis SemiSerif Pro by Jouve (UK), Milton Keynes
Printed and bound in Great Britain by Clays Ltd, Elcograf S.p.A.

The authorised representative in the EEA is Penguin Random House Ireland,
Morrison Chambers, 32 Nassau Street, Dublin D02 YH68

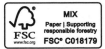

MIX
Paper | Supporting
responsible forestry
FSC® C018179

Penguin Random House is committed
to a sustainable future for our business,
our readers and our planet. This book is
made from Forest Stewardship Council®
certified paper.

'I've always been a big believer in the magic of creativity.'

– Olivia Rodrigo

CONTENTS

INTRODUCTION

Livies know that Olivia Rodrigo's words of wisdom are the perfect guide for thriving in today's crazy world.

Releasing 'Driver's License' while still a teenager, Olivia Rodrigo has experienced a meteoric rise to global fame. She has won numerous awards and has been named *Time*'s Entertainer of the Year, *Billboard*'s Woman of the Year and Songwriter of the Year by *Variety*. Quite frankly, we're obsessed.

Olivia has met President Biden and performed at Glastonbury. Yet, through all this, she has stayed grounded and true to herself. So, what are her secrets? Find out what Olivia thinks about growing up, creativity, resilience, friendship and having fun. Dive in – it'll be Good 4 U.

From being home-schooled and an actor at such a young age, Olivia knows what it's like to forge your own path. In these pages, she explains her fierce work ethic and exactly what it takes to make it, and stay happier. Turn to Olivia's wisdom if you need words of advice, support to pursue your dreams and help to deal with your real big mistakes.

When not song-writing, performing and making friends with megastars like Billie Eilish and Selena Gomez, Olivia finds time to be a fierce advocate for women using her platform to raise awareness of the issues she cares about. The inspiring advice in this book will give you the guts to live the life you deserve.

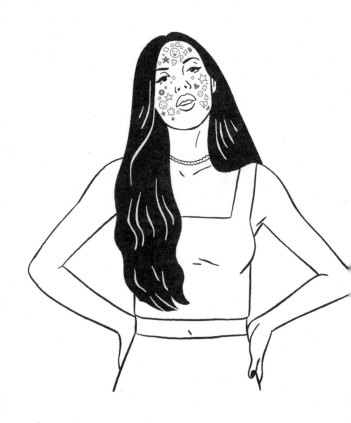

EMOTIONS

'I'm just obsessed with emotions. I'm the most sensitive bitch in the whole world.'

'I love nineties girls who aren't afraid to be angry and remorseful and like spiteful and snarling.'

'Women are so discouraged from showing emotions, like anger or dissatisfaction for fear of being ungrateful or hard to be around, and I've always struggled with that.'

'I've always admired women that are really vulnerable and honest in their music, it's a hard thing to do. And, you know, all of my idols do that.'

'... this repressed anger and confusion of being put into a box as a girl.'

'It's nice to kind of look back at issues that I thought were gonna be world-ending and be like, "Ah, that worked out, totally fine. It made me who I am".'

'Lots of my songs are literally about crying, which is very Pisces, but I'm a little angsty, too.'

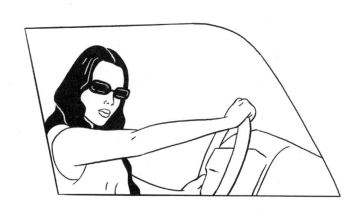

GROWING UP

'I remember when I was like, 13, and they were asking me what I wanted my brand to be, and I was just like, I don't even know what I want to wear tomorrow.'

'You don't realize
how young you are,
when you're young.'

'I feel like I am
ever changing,
ever evolving.'

'I'm so happy
to be a girl.'

'I've always struggled with wanting to be this perfect American girl and the reality of not feeling like that all the time.'

'I love my generation.
I am proud to be
a part of it.'

'We undersell how
full of rage and angst
young people are.'

'I was a child actor
when I was young.
I was very driven
and really wanted
to succeed.'

'I feel like you need a little delusion to get by. It's just, hope, you know, another word for positive attitude.'

'February is my favourite
month because it's
my birthday.'

'Gen Z in particular has such a bulls – barometer. We want to know what's behind everything.'

'It's going to
work out.'

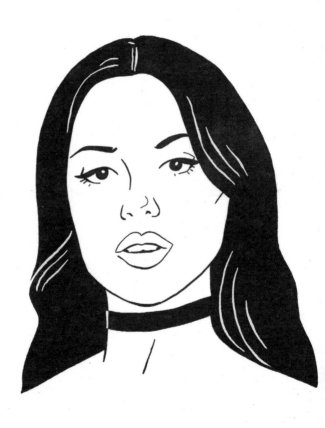

CREATIVITY

'I do believe that creativity sometimes is kind of something beyond you. It's like a magic that we as humans with egos can't control.'

'Sprinkle of this,
sprinkle of that.'

'Write the songs
of your heart.'

'I love using a swearword when it's tasteful and necessary.'

'I feel like every song
I've ever written is just
me spilling my guts
a little bit.'

'Writing songs will hopefully always be an outlet for me to process my feelings before anything else.'

'Every single artist
is inspired by artists
who have come before
them. It's sort of a fun,
beautiful sharing process.
Nothing in music is ever
new. There's four chords
in every song. That's
the fun part – trying to
make that your own.'

'When you have every colour in the palette and any canvas you want, it's just so overwhelming that sometimes I think limiting yourself actually makes you think outside the box and reinvent.'

'That's what's beautiful about art – you can just fill in the gaps with pieces of your own life.'

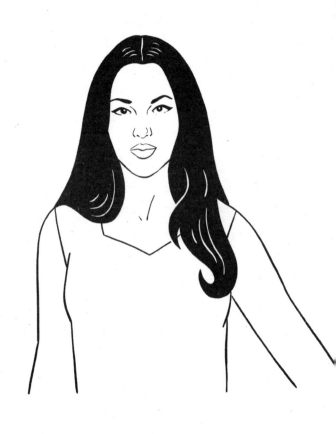

WORK
ETHIC

'I try to write
every day.'

'You definitely have to
be a businesswoman
to be a musician.'

'I think showing up is really important. It's more important than being talented or good at anything because you can be super talented, but if you don't show up, what's the point?'

'Sometimes, you [. . .] have a lightning bolt idea and you can write one song in 30 minutes. But it's not about those 30 minutes; it's about the hundreds of songs you write before that to practise for a 30-minute song.'

'Just believe in yourself
and keep trying.'

'Song names, concepts, lyrics just come randomly throughout the day in your normal life. I'll just write them down, the trick is having the work ethic + focus to flesh it out + make it into something.'

'We definitely had some tricky moments where we were like, "How are we gonna do this? Are we good at this?" We actually coined a term for it when we were in the studio and we were doing really bad, we called it the dread.'

'I'm a big believer in creativity as a discipline.'

'Never give up.'

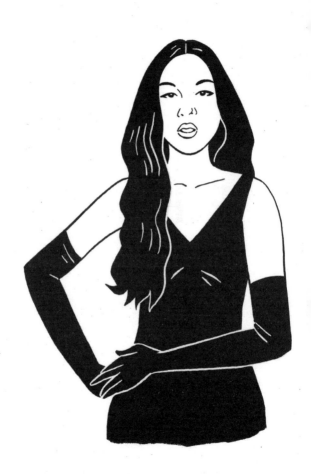

FEMINISM

'People talk about women's bodies in a way that's completely unjust.'

'I guess the first song that I wrote on piano, proper, I was probably 14 or 15, and I wrote this feminist anthem called "Superman," about how I didn't need Superman to come and save me. Start them young.'

'I don't really subscribe to hating other women because of boys. I think that's so stupid.'

'The Supreme Court decided to overturn Roe v Wade, which is the law that ensures a woman's right to a safe abortion, and other basic human rights. I'm devastated and terrified that so many women and so many girls are going to die because of this.'

'Young women are constantly compared to each other ... and that can be reductive.'

'It's unhealthy for young girls to be looking at all that stuff in the media. It paints a bad picture.'

'I really love women who are not afraid to speak their mind and tell their perspective.'

'I kind of felt this pressure to be this girl that I thought everyone expected me to be.'

'You have the power
to save lives.'

'It would be a bald-faced lie if I say that I didn't face any misogyny in the music industry – especially being a young girl.'

'We all need to keep speaking out against these injustices in the world.'

'It's so exciting to me to watch young women's voices be heard and appreciated and celebrated.'

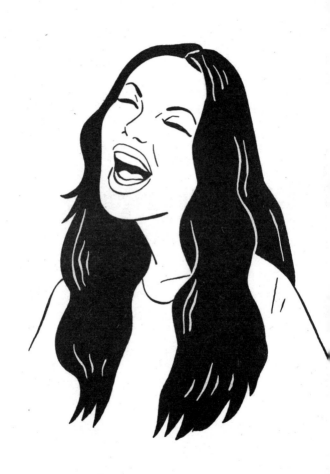

FRIENDSHIP

'I feel so lucky that I just like was born at the right time to be able to look up to somebody like [Taylor Swift].'

'I think [Taylor is] the best songwriter of all time, but she's so business-savvy and she really cares about her career in that regard too – that's been really inspiring for me to watch somebody take control of their career and their life like that.'

'I love Kelly Clarkson
and I grew up
listening to her.'

'And [Phoebe Bridgers is] just the coolest person in the world and her music's so great.'

'[Elizabeth Gilbert] has this whole chapter about how the starving artist complex is like, stupid, essentially. And how, if you're a fulfilled, happy person, your art can only be more whole and better received. So I like to subscribe to that mindset.'

'[Billie Eilish is] so intelligent and I think it's so awesome that girls can look up to somebody like her.'

'[Selena Gomez] was so kind. She talked to me a lot about prioritizing mental health, which I think is really important in this industry. All of us were in the limelight very young. . . . That can be taxing on your psyche and can bring about all these weird issues.'

'Alanis [Morissette],
you're a trailblazer
and you have inspired
an entire generation
of uncompromising,
radically honest
songwriting.'

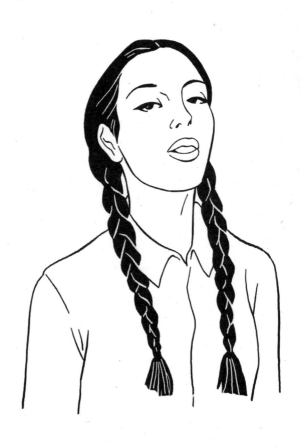

HAVING FUN

'Hang out with
your best friends.'

'We scream at the top of our lungs and dance in our [car] seats.'

Interviewer: What's your style?

Olivia: Vibes.

'Any time I'm stressed out, I just get in the car and drive around aimlessly and listen to music or something.'

'I would love to say bad idea, but that sounds like so much fun.'

'Rolling down a hill, there's nothing quite like it, there's no greater experience of joy.'

'You deserve a rest.
Take a bubble bath.'

'Ah so much
drama!'

'Every day of my life I
try to be more and more
like Carrie Bradshaw.'

'Last night I had peanut M&Ms for dinner.'

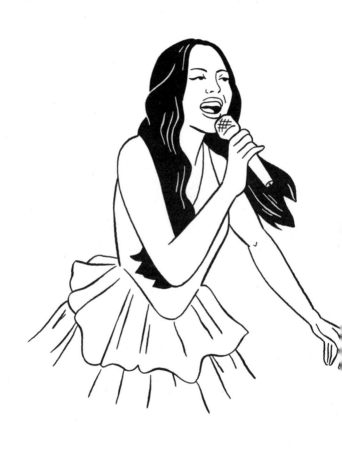

LOVE

'I literally wrote breakup songs before I'd ever held a boy's hand or even remotely dated someone.'

'Maybe I did things that maybe I shouldn't have – dated people that I shouldn't have.'

'We're all so much more alike than we are different. At the core of every human is the same feeling of love and anger and heartbreak.'

'Heartbreak is a
two-way street.'

'I think all the songs are sort of a different aspect of heartbreak. There's plenty of emotions that come along with something like that: anger, spite, sadness, jealousy, longing.'

'Long-distance relationships are so hard. That stuff is hard.'

'I think heartbreak is so universal – the feeling that lots of humans feel the most deeply.'

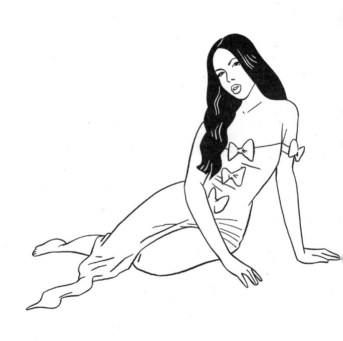

RESILIENCE

'If I'm ever stressed out,
I like jump in a pool,
or ocean, even going
in the shower, and I'm
just reborn.'

'I realised . . . that I
would rather spend time
with myself than people
who make me weary
or cause me anxiety or
drag me down.'

'At the end of the day, making mistakes is the only way you do learn.'

'I feel like the more you try to control it, the more miserable you are, and the bigger it gets.'

'I'm trying not to pretend like I have everything figured out because I sure as hell don't.'

'I felt a little lost, but
I stuck with it, and I
kind of had to shift
my mindset.'

'Put your horseblinders
on and focus on what
you can control.'

'Taking responsibility for my mental health and sanity has been a really important lesson that I had to learn throughout all of this . . . it's so easy to get fucked up in all of the craziness of the industry.'

'I have many blessings
in my life, but my life is
definitely not perfect.'

'Many times people associate vulnerability with weakness. From a young age, I realised that vulnerability equates to strength.'

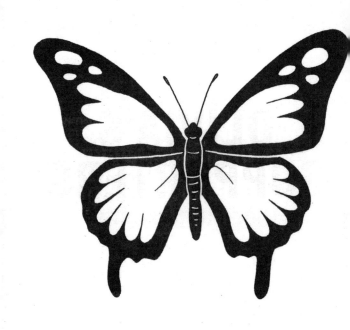

OLIVIA'S
SUPPORTERS

'I say that's my baby
and I'm really proud.'

– Taylor Swift

'She's the real deal.
She's precious.'

– Sheryl Crow

'She's never satisfied. With Olivia . . . there's a constant, like, "What if we tried this? What if we changed all the pianos out and made them guitars? What if we rewrote the lyrics?" No song feels like it's done.'

– Dan Nigro

'I think it's important for people like Olivia to give an honest voice to so many young women who are still discovering themselves. Her songs are her truth, and you can really feel that.'

– Avril Lavigne

'A gift of knowing how to tell a story in a song.'

– Carole King

'She has a steadfast care about self-expression. She's not precious about it, nor does she seem overwhelmed by it all.'

– Alanis Morissette

'I think she's a really amazing artist and I love so many of the songs she's released . . . so honest, so vulnerable.'

– Camila Cabello

'It's always cool to be compared to an artist that is so big and amazing, and somebody that everybody looks up to right now.'

– Mckenna Grace

'Nobody has had anybody else's life, you know? But I do feel a protectiveness over Olivia.'

– Billie Eilish

'I think it's kind of a cool thing to introduce the whole generation of young people to different musical ideas.'

– Adam Levine

ACKNOWLEDGEMENTS

Page 6 from Interview, 'For Olivia Rodrigo, "Drivers License" Is Only the Beginning' (Ben Barna, 2021). Page 7 from Hits Radio, 'For The Record – Olivia Rodrigo breaks down 'Vampire' and new album 'Guts' (2023). Page 8 from BBC news, 'Olivia Rodrigo interview: 'I've got a few heartbreaks left in me'' (Mark Savage, 2023). Page 9 from Music Week, 'Olivia Rodrigo on songwriting and vulnerability, the meaning behind her lyrics & Sour's huge success' (Anna Fielding, 2021).Page 10 from Apple Music, The Zane Lowe Show (2023). Page 11 from GQ, '10 things Olivia Rodrigo Can't Live Without' (2023). Page 12 from Clash, 'Living Her Teenage Dream: Olivia Rodrigo Interviewed', (Ilana Kaplan, 2021). Page 16 from from US Vogue.com, 'A New Decade, A New Album, A New Life—Olivia Rodrigo's Next Chapter' (Jia Tolentino, 2023). Page 17 from US Vogue.com, 'A New Decade, A New Album, A New Life—Olivia Rodrigo's Next Chapter' (Jia Tolentino, 2023). Page 18 from Wired, 'Olivia Rodrigo Answers The Web's Most Searched Questions' (2023). Page 19 from Rolling Stone, 'Olivia Rodrigo Is So Over Heartbreak' (Angie Martoccio, 2023).Page 20 from The Guardian, "I had all these feelings of rage I couldn't express': Olivia Rodrigo on overnight pop superstardom, plagiarism and growing up in public" (Laura Snapes, 2023). Page 21 from The New Yorker, 'Olivia Rodrigo on the Meanings of "Guts"' (David Remnick, 2023). Page 22 from Interview, 'Olivia Rodrigo and Phoebe Bridgers Let It All Out' (Phoebe Bridgers, 2023). Page 23 from The Hollywood Reporter, ''Awards Chatter' Podcast – Olivia Rodrigo (Scott Feinberg, 2023). Page 24 from Sirius XM, TikTok Radio IRL – Olivia Rodrigo on 'GUTS' Album, Having a Hot Girl Summer, Living in New York City' (Davis Burleson, 2023). Page 25 from The Late Late Show, 23 March 22. Page 26 from Los Angeles Times, 'How Olivia Rodrigo went from Disney princess to pop queen' (Mikael Wood, 2021). Page 27 from Sirius XM, TikTok Radio IRL – Olivia Rodrigo on 'GUTS' Album, Having a Hot Girl Summer, Living in New York City' (Davis Burleson, 2023).Page 30 from The New Yorker, 'Olivia Rodrigo on the Meanings of "Guts"' (David Remnick, 2023). Page 31 from Sirius XM, TikTok Radio IRL – Olivia Rodrigo on 'GUTS' Album, Having a Hot Girl Summer, Living in New York City' (Davis Burleson, 2023). Page 32 from GQ, '10 things Olivia Rodrigo Can't Live Without' (2023). Page 33 from Jimmy Kimmel Live! 24 Oct 23. Page 34 from Sunday Today with Willie Geist, 10 September 2023. Page 35 from Billboard, 'Woman Of The Year Olivia Rodrigo Is Writing New Music (And Reuniting With A Big Collaborator)' (Andrew Unterberger, 2023). Page 36 from Teen Vogue, 'Olivia Rodrigo at the Crossroads' (P. Claire Dodson, 2021). Page 37 from The Hollywood Reporter, 'The Hit Squad: Billie Eilish, Olivia Rodrigo and

ACKNOWLEDGEMENTS

Dua Lipa on the THR Songwriter Roundtable' (Mesfin Fekadu, 2023). Page 38 from Rolling Stone, 'Musicians on Musicians: Alanis Morissette & Olivia Rodrigo' (Angie Martoccio, 2021). Page 42 from Rolling Stone, 'Musicians on Musicians: Alanis Morissette & Olivia Rodrigo' (Angie Martoccio, 2021). Page 43 from Time, 'Entertainer of the Year' (Lucy Feldman, 2021). Page 44 from MTV News, 'Olivia Rodrigo on Her Top 5 Songwriting Tips' (2021). Page 45 from Vogue Singapore, 'Olivia Rodrigo on her upward trajectory to fame, being part of Gen Z and keeping her mental health in check' (Amelia Chia, 2021). Page 46 from Vogue, '73 Questions with Olivia Rodrigo' (Joe Sabia, 2023). Page 47 from GQ, Actually Me – Olivia Rodrigo Replies to Fans on the Internet (2021). Page 48 from US magazine, 'Olivia Rodrigo jokes she 'tortured' her cowriter over decisions about Guts' lead single' (Shelby Stivale, 2023). Page 49 from Teen Vogue, 'Olivia Rodrigo at the Crossroads' (P. Claire Dodson, 2021). Page 50 from Apple Music, The Zane Lowe Show (2023).Page 54 from from Los Angeles Times, 'How Olivia Rodrigo went from Disney princess to pop queen' (Mikael Wood, 2021). Page 55 from The Hollywood Reporter, 'The Hit Squad: Billie Eilish, Olivia Rodrigo and Dua Lipa on the THR Songwriter Roundtable' (Mesfin Fekadu, 2023). Page 56 from Variety, 'From Disney to 'Drivers License': Inside Olivia Rodrigo's Musical Journey to Become the Voice of Her Generation' (Ellise Shafer, 2021). Page 57 from British Vogue, 'Olivia Rodrigo's Glastonbury Set Came With A Powerful Roe V Wade Message' (Liam Hess, 2022). Page 58 from Time, 'Entertainer of the Year' (Lucy Feldman, 2021). Page 59 from Teen Vogue, 'Olivia Rodrigo at the Crossroads' (P. Claire Dodson, 2021). Page 60 from Clash, 'Living Her Teenage Dream: Olivia Rodrigo Interviewed' (Ilana Kaplan, 2021). Page 61 from Los Angeles Times, 'Bad idea, right? Olivia Rodrigo says she dated people she 'shouldn't have' after 'Sour'' (Christi Carras, 2023). Page 62 from Instagram, 15 July 2021. Page 63 from NME, 'Olivia Rodrigo: "It's important for me to be taken seriously as a songwriter"' (Hannah Mylrea, 2021). Page 64 from Billboard, 'License To Thrive: Olivia Rodrigo Zooms Ahead After 2021's Biggest Breakout Hit' (Andrew Unterberger, 2021). Page 65 from Billboard, 'Woman Of The Year Olivia Rodrigo Is Writing New Music (And Reuniting With A Big Collaborator)' (Andrew Unterberger, 2023). Page 68 from SiriusXM, 'Taylor Swift Sent Olivia Rodrigo a Really Special Gift' (2021). Page 69 from NME, 'Olivia Rodrigo: "It's important for me to be taken seriously as a songwriter"' (Hannah Mylrea, 2021). Page 70 from GQ, 'Actually Me – Olivia Rodrigo Replies to Fans on the Internet' (2021). Page 71 from Elle, 'Is This the End of Olivia Rodrigo's Sad Girl Era?' (Erica Gonzales, 2022). Page 72 from Elle, 'Is This the End of Olivia Rodrigo's Sad Girl Era?' (Erica Gonzales, 2022). Page 73 from NME, 'Olivia Rodrigo: "It's important for me to be taken seriously as a songwriter"' (Hannah Mylrea, 2021). Page 74 from Variety, 'From Disney to 'Drivers License': Inside Olivia Rodrigo's Musical Journey to Become the Voice of Her Generation' (Ellise Shafer, 2021). Page 75 from Canadian Songwriters Hall of Fame, 'Olivia Rodrigo Inducts Alanis Morissette into the Canadian Songwriters Hall of Fame' (2023). Page 78 from Seventeen.com , '7 Questions: Olivia Rodrigo Shares Her Favorite Lyrics on 'SOUR,' The Best Way To Get Over a Breakup' (Samantha Olson, 2021). Page 79 from Seventeen.com , '7 Questions: Olivia Rodrigo Shares Her Favorite Lyrics on 'SOUR,' The Best Way To Get Over a Breakup' (Samantha Olson, 2021). Page 80 from Time, 'Entertainer of the Year' (Lucy Feldman, 2021). Page 81 from Billboard, 'License To Thrive: Olivia Rodrigo Zooms Ahead After 2021's Biggest

ACKNOWLEDGEMENTS

Breakout Hit' (Andrew Unterberger, 2021). Page 83 from Capital FM, 'Olivia Rodrigo rates British things (2023). Page 84 from Interview, 'Olivia Rodrigo and Phoebe Bridgers Let It All Out' (Phoebe Bridgers, 2023). Page 85 from PopBuzz, 'Olivia Rodrigo vs. 'The Most Impossible Olivia Rodrigo Quiz'' (2023). Page 86 from Vogue, '73 Questions with Olivia Rodrigo' (Joe Sabia, 2023). Page 87 from The Late Late Show, 23 March 22. Page 90 from Variety, 'From Disney to 'Drivers License': Inside Olivia Rodrigo's Musical Journey to Become the Voice of Her Generation' (Ellise Shafer, 2021). Page 91 from Los Angeles Times, 'Bad idea, right? Olivia Rodrigo says she dated people she 'shouldn't have' after 'Sour'' (Christi Carras, 2023). Page 92 from BBC news, 'Olivia Rodrigo interview: 'I've got a few heartbreaks left in me'' (Mark Savage 2023).Page 93 from Elle, Is This the End of Olivia Rodrigo's Sad Girl Era?' (Erica Gonzales, 2022). Page 94 from Variety, 'From Disney to 'Drivers License': Inside Olivia Rodrigo's Musical Journey to Become the Voice of Her Generation' (Ellise Shafer, 2021). Page 95 from Seventeen.com , '7 Questions: Olivia Rodrigo Shares Her Favorite Lyrics on 'SOUR,' The Best Way To Get Over a Breakup' (Samantha Olson, 2021). Page 96 from Rolling Stone, 'Musicians on Musicians: Alanis Morissette & Olivia Rodrigo' (Angie Martoccio, 2021). Page 100 from Wired, 'Olivia Rodrigo Answers The Web's Most Searched Questions' (2023). Page 101 from The Guardian, ''I had all these feelings of rage I couldn't express': Olivia Rodrigo on overnight pop superstardom, plagiarism and growing up in public'' (Laura Snapes, 2023). Page 102 from The New Yorker, 'Olivia Rodrigo on the Meanings of "Guts"' (David Remnick, 2023). Page 103 from Rolling Stone, 'Musicians on Musicians: Alanis Morissette & Olivia Rodrigo' (Angie Martoccio, 2021). Page 104 from Interview, 'For Olivia Rodrigo, "Drivers License" Is Only the Beginning' (Ben Barna, 2021). Page 105 from from Hits Radio, 'For The Record – Olivia Rodrigo breaks down 'Vampire' and new album 'Guts' (2023). Page 106 from Sunday Today with Willie Geist, 10 September 2023. Page 107 from Clash, 'Living Her Teenage Dream: Olivia Rodrigo Interviewed, (Ilana Kaplan, 2021). Page 108 from GQ, Actually Me - Olivia Rodrigo Replies to Fans on the Internet (2021). Page 109 from Vogue Singapore, 'Olivia Rodrigo on her upward trajectory to fame, being part of Gen Z and keeping her mental health in check' (Amelia Chia, 2021). Page 112 from Elle Australia, 'The Full Timeline Of Taylor Swift And Olivia Rodrigo's Alleged Feud' (2023). Page 113 from The Tonight Show Starring Jimmy Fallon , 3 November 2023. Page 114 from Billboard, 'License To Thrive: Olivia Rodrigo Zooms Ahead After 2021's Biggest Breakout Hit' (Andrew Unterberger, 2021). Page 115 from Variety, 'From Disney to 'Drivers License': Inside Olivia Rodrigo's Musical Journey to Become the Voice of Her Generation' (Ellise Shafer, 2021). Page 116 from Time, 'Entertainer of the Year' (Lucy Feldman, 2021). Page 117 from Time, 'Entertainer of the Year' (Lucy Feldman, 2021). Page 118 from BBC, Radio 1's Live Lounge, 7th September 2021. Page 119 from Paper, 'Mckenna Grace's Sad Girl Era Is Upon Us'(Bailer Richards, 2022). Page 120 from Los Angeles Times, 'What Billie Eilish learned from her own Barbie song "What Was I made for?"' (Mikael Wood, 2023). Page 121 from Los Angeles Times, 'Adam Levine shows compassion for Olivia Rodrigo amid plagiarism claims' (Christi Carras, 2021).